PLAYING SAFE ALWAYS:

Being in control when your best friend has borderline personality disorder

By

Wendy C. Watson

Table of contents

INTRODUCTION

This book gives you knowledge of how Individuals with BPD attempt to deal with their aggravation through their associations with others. projections, seethes, analysis, accusing, and other safeguard components might be endeavors to inspire you to sympathize with their aggravation for them. At the point when you emphatically divert the aggravation back to the individual with BPD so they can start to manage it, you are breaking an agreement that you didn't realize you marked. Normally, the individual with BPD will view this as troubling. The individual with BPD will likely make a countermove. This is an activity intended to reestablish things to how they were. Countermoves additionally assist individuals with legitimizing their activities, both to themselves and to you. This component is pivotal because it appears to make the shakedown satisfactory — even honorable. Your capacity to endure these countermoves will decide the future course of your relationship. This will assist you with dealing with your closest companions' BPD without getting injured yourself.

Playing safe always

CHAPTER 1

Do you know someone who has narcissistic or borderline personality disorder?

Narcissism (more precisely, narcissistic personality disorder, or NPD) and borderline personality disorder are both types of personality disorders. The symptoms of one condition may grow worse when the two coexist. The disorders may be more difficult to diagnose and cure. Yet, it's conceivable that treating BPD (borderline personality disorder) might help lessen some of the NPD symptoms.
Dysfunction of the narcissistic personality (NPD)
Five or more of the following symptoms must be present to be diagnosed with narcissistic personality disorder:

- feeling of entitlement
- self-importance that is exaggerated
- Strange, self-obsessed, or boastful actions

- Having envy for others or thinking that others have envy of them
- Absence of empathy
- obsession with prosperity, dominance, brilliance, attractiveness, or ideal love fantasies
- excessive adoration required
- Exploiting others
- Thinking they are "special" and can only be understood by other exceptional or high-status individuals.

Simply put, those who have NPD are often exceedingly egocentric or self-absorbed. Whenever a person's alliances, career, or other critical areas of their life are adversely impacted, their self-absorption becomes severe enough to qualify as a psychiatric condition. According to many experts, this egocentric behavior is essentially an effort to address underlying esteem. Dysfunction of the Borderline Personality (BPD).

Furthermore, a Cluster B personality disorder, borderline personality disorder (BPD) is one. It is distinguished by continuous shifts in behavior, attitude, and personality. Anger, depression, and panic crises that last a few days or longer are frequent among BPD sufferers.

BPD sufferers regularly alter their perspectives on another, themselves, and their hobbies. Friendships and relationships are frequently turbulent or unpredictable when there are significant shifts in viewpoint. Additional BPD clinical manifestations include:

- severe dread of being abandoned
- Impetuous actions (such as unsafe sex or substance use)
- Self-harm
- Suicide-related thoughts

Dissociation is a symptom that BPD sufferers may experience, particularly under stress. Dissociation can make a person feel as though they are losing their sense of belonging or self. They could feel cut off from their feelings, experiences, and ideas. Also, they may lose a lot of recollection about certain events, individuals, and seasons in their lives. It can be challenging to distinguish between borderline personality disorder (BPD) and narcissistic personality disorder (NPD) in a close friendship since their symptoms might overlap.

You may decide how to alter the circumstances in your relationship by being aware of the variations between violent relationships with BPD and NPD. There are tools available to assist you in protecting yourself from an abusive spouse or ending a violent relationship, irrespective of an underlying anxiety or depression is present. Abusive behavior is a decision, and it is never acceptable.

Thoughts and conduct can change quickly in people with borderline personality disorder (BPD), specifically whenever they feel intimidated by rejection.

These signs usually involve:
- great precautions to prevent desertion
- erratic sense of self-identity
- a pattern of unhappy relationships
- irresponsibility in at minimum two instances of self-destructive conduct, such as unusually large amounts of food, overspending, or abusing drugs and alcohol persistent
- sense of loneliness
- difficulties managing excessive or extreme anger

- hallucination brought on by stress or signs of detachment

In general, a person must exhibit at least five of these characteristics or more to be diagnosed with BPD. Individuals that have NPD are frequently perceived as someone being self-centered and believing that they are superior to or higher than some other individuals. Yet the disorder is far more complex than that. NPD sufferers may also struggle to comprehend other people's feelings and motivations. NPD is diagnosed when a person exhibits at least five of the symptoms listed below:

Symptoms of BPD versus NPD

By looking at the actions and reasons behind the manifestations, such as temper tantrums, it is simpler to distinguish between the two illnesses.

Intentions for conduct

Deception (possibly rudeness) (potentially verbally abusive)

NPD: manipulates people to preserve the sense of significance by dismissing and depreciating them

BPD tries to prevent rejection by manipulating others through jealousy, threats (particularly self-harm), or domination.

A confrontation with their feeling of self-importance makes **NPD** angry.

BPD: is more detached and emotionally vulnerable, making them unable to understand the viewpoints of others.

recurrent voidness or nothingness

emotionally vapid according to **NPD**

BPD: Has strong emotions of rejection

sensitivity to emotion

Admires their target, cheapens them, and ultimately discards them according to **NPD**.

BPD: exhibits affection but then switches to wrath, fear, or contempt to prevent rejection

lacking in empathy

A continuous lack of compassion is displayed by **NPD**.

BPD: Depending on their emotional state, they either exhibit genuine compassion or a lack of it. Borderline personality disorder (BPD) and personality disorder (NPD) are two mental health illnesses that are sometimes confused with one another because they have some similar characteristics. These diseases fall under the umbrella of cluster B personality disorders, which are distinguished by excessively emotional or unpredictable thoughts or behavior.

It's crucial to keep in mind while contrasting narcissism with a borderline personality disorder that, despite having some similar symptoms, each illness is unique and has its own set of diagnosis requirements. For instance, both diseases have inappropriate ways of handling conflicts that are harmful to both the people around them and themselves. Yet, how conflict-related rage is expressed differs.

The Connection Between BPD and NPD

In addition to co-occurring borderline personality disorder, a narcissistic personality disorder can also thrive on its own. Understanding the connection between BPD and NPD is essential in ascertaining that certain indicators of the two diseases are similar. An individual who struggles in daily life will result from combining the characteristics of NPD with BPD.

Another connection between narcissism and borderline personality disorder is that both NPD and BPD sufferers battle a crippling history of anxiety. The difficulty of staying in touch with others amid these illnesses adds to the dread of loss. In fact, "deep and turbulent relationships" is one of BPD's defining characteristics.

That second component is just absent in the narcissist's reality. Narcissists are unable to look beyond themselves and take into account what others may think. This has an impact on someone with NPD's mental-interpersonal functioning, as well as their capacity to sustain relationships.

Yet, BPD sufferers frequently overreact to other people's worries, particularly during the period known as the "idealization" stage of a relationship. But, placing one another's needs above your own will ultimately lead to anger and resentment cycles that cause resentment, and at that time the connection will enter the "depreciation" stage.

CHAPTER 2

Borderline personality disorder explanation

A problem of temperament and social interaction is known as a borderline personality disorder (BPD). The far more prevalent personality disorder is this one.

Generally speaking, a person with a personality disorder will behave very differently from the ordinary individual in the sense of how they think, interpret, experience, and react to others.

Borderline personality disorder signs and symptoms (BPD)

Four major categories of BPD symptoms include: Emotional turbulence is the clinical explanation for mental instability. disrupted thought or perception processes, such as cognition abnormalities

Impulsive behavior strong yet erratic interpersonal interactions

A personality disorder often manifests in youth and lasts throughout adulthood. The symptoms can range from moderate to severe.

Borderline personality disorder causes (BPD)

BPD's origins are unknown. It indicates that a mix of hereditary and environmental variables contribute to BPD.

BPD sufferers come from a variety of experiences, but most will have been subjected to the trauma of some form or have suffered abandonment by loved ones.

Most BPD sufferers eventually get well and conquer psychological symptoms. Those whose problems reoccur are advised to seek further therapy. Even if you have a borderline personality disorder (BPD), you may have unpredictable moods, unhealthy relationships, and a shaky understanding of who you are. As a result, you may feel like you're already on a Ferris wheel. Your objectives, self-perception, and even your preferences may fluctuate regularly which seems hazy and imprecise.

BPD sufferers are frequently very sensitive. Some compare it to having a sensory terminal uncovered. Tremendous responses can be brought on by simple details. You also have a hard time defrosting once you're agitated. It is simple to see how this emotional state and impaired functioning with one's feelings cause problems in relationships and aggressive, even dangerous, conduct.

Whenever you're experiencing extreme feelings, it's difficult to remain rational or focused. You could produce nasty remarks or behave in risky or improper ways, which will help you feel bad or humiliated thereafter. It's a vicious circle from which it may seem hard to break free. Yet it isn't. You may feel happier and regain a sense of your emotions, moods, and behavior with the use of BPD therapies and resilience. Borderline personality disorder (BPD) was formerly refractory to treatment, leading many psychiatrists and psychologists to believe that there wasn't much that could be performed. Nonetheless, we now understand that BPD is curable. In actuality, BPD has a decent long outlook than both bipolar disorders and depressive disorders. Nonetheless, it necessitates a unique strategy. The majority of BPD sufferers are capable of recovering, and with the correct assistance and therapies, they do so rather quickly. Eliminating the unhealthy thought, feelings, and behavior patterns that are giving you pain are the first step in recovering. It's difficult to break ingrained behaviors. Initially, deciding to halt, think, and then take new actions will seem strange. Yet as time passes, you'll develop new routines that assist you in keeping your emotions in check and remaining in charge.

Borderline personality disorder recognition

Do the following statements apply to you?

I frequently feel "empty."

I face enormous despair, rage, and worry rather frequently, and my feelings change quite fast.

I live in continual fear that the individuals that I care about will depart or forsake me.

The majority of my romances would be considered passionate yet unpredictable.

I do not often comprehend why my feelings for the individuals who exist in my life may fluctuate drastically from one instant to the next.

I frequently engage in behaviors that I am aware to be risky or harmful, such as speeding carelessly, engaging in risky sexual activity, alcohol consumption, abusing drugs, or engaging in shopping binges.

I have made attempts to damage myself, slashed myself, or verbally assaulted myself.

I often lash out or act rashly in relationships when I'm insecure in attempting to maintain the other individual near me.

The nine signs of BPD

- **A dread of rejection.** A common fear of BPD sufferers is being discarded or left lonely. Even seemingly little events, such as close ones leaving for the weekends or coming back from the office late, can cause extreme panic. This may result in desperate attempts to hold the other person near. You could nag, cling, pick conflicts, follow the whereabouts of your loved one, or even violently prohibit them from exiting. However, this action frequently has the reverse effect alienating other people.

- **Fragile connections.** Strong and transient relationships are more prevalent in persons with BPD. You could find love rapidly, thinking that every stranger would complete you, and then be turned down right away. There is no invincibility in your relationships—either they are good or they are bad for it can neither be lukewarm. Your fast fluctuations from the idealized version to depreciation, wrath, and hate may leave your partners, acquaintances, or close relatives experiencing psychological instability.

- **A vague or changing notion of oneself.** Your self-worth is often shaky during BPD. You could occasionally feel positive regarding yourself, although in other instances you could perhaps detest or despise yourself. Most likely, you are unsure of your identity and whatever you desire from your existence. You could as a result regularly switch between professions, acquaintances, partners, religions, values, and even sexual identities.

- **Self-destructive, uncontrolled actions.** Once you're unhappy, especially if you have BPD, you could act in dangerous, pleasurable ways. You could overindulge in illegal substances, have excessive food, drive dangerously, shoplift, participate in unsafe sex, or waste cash you probably couldn't afford to. While engaging in these dangerous habits may improve your state of mind at the time, elsewhere in the big scheme of things, they are bad for both you and the people closest to you.

- **Consciousness, Individuals with BPD frequently engage in intentional self-harm and homicidal conduct.** Suicide attempts conduct involves building in you some suicide thoughts signals or attempts, thinking of suicide, and going forward to actualize the thought to commit suicide. Any other attempts to damage yourself without a suicide motive are considered self-harm. Self-harm techniques including setting fires are often used.

- **Dramatic mood changes.** In BPD, unpredictable emotional states are frequent. You can feel happy one point in time and downcasted the next. You may become emotionally distraught about seemingly insignificant issues that others choose to ignore. Unlike the hormonal fluctuations of depression and anxiety or bipolar disease, these hormonal changes are severe but often dissipate rapidly, lasting only a few seconds or minutes.

- **Persistent loneliness in the heart.** Individuals who have BPD frequently describe feeling as though they have a hole or vacuum inside of them. At your worst, you could feel like "nothing" or "nobody." You can attempt to replace the unpleasant sensation with substances like food, sex, or narcotics. Nevertheless, nothing is gratifying.

- **Furious rage.** If you have BPD, you can have trouble controlling your extreme wrath and fury. After the fuse is ignited, you can also lose control and lose control of yourself, shouting, throwing objects, or losing control of your anger altogether. It's important to notice that not all of this anger has an external focus. You can find yourself unnecessary getting upset with yourself on a daily basis.

- **Sense of unreliability or suspicion.** Individuals with BPD frequently deal with anxiety or questions about the motivations of everyone else. You could even lose contact with the outside world while being under duress, a condition known as detachment. You could experience blurriness, fuzziness, or a sense of being outside of your body.

To put it simply, your brain is a hyper-alert if you have BPD. You may experience more anxiety and fear than other individuals. The grudge match circuit is quickly triggered, and once it does, it takes over your logical mind and activates instincts for survival that aren't necessarily suitable for the current circumstance.

This may give the impression that there isn't anything you can do. After all, if the thinking is distinct, what would you do? But, the reality is how you can alter your intellect. You build new brain connections each time you employ a new coping mechanism or self-calming strategy. Certain therapies, including relaxation techniques, can even stimulate the growth of new brain tissue. And these routes will get better and much more spontaneous the further you train. So keep trying! You are capable of altering your thoughts, feelings, and behaviors with effort and time.

When psychologists use the word "personality," they're alluding to the distinctive ways that each of us thought, feel, and act. While no one behaves precisely these all the time, we do tend to participate in similar interactions and activities with the outside world. Because of this, persons are frequently referred to be "quiet," "extroverted," "careful," "enjoyable," etc. Certain character traits are present.

The phrase "personality disorder" may make you feel as though there is nothing profoundly wrong with your character since personality and sense of self are so closely related. A personality disorder, however, is not a moral assessment. Your style of connecting to the outside world is markedly unique and different, which is what "personality disorder" indicates in professional words. You don't behave in a way that some people would anticipate, differently in different words. Your relationships, job, and self-esteem are all negatively impacted by this, and it also negatively affects how you perceive other people.

The far more crucial thing is that these designs may be altered! When tension starts to get the better of you, you may relax by using the relaxing strategies we've already covered. But what should you see if you're experiencing a wave of distressing emotions? This is where borderline personality disorder (BPD impulsivity)'s enters the picture. You're extremely eager for relief inside the moment's tense circumstances that you'll do whatever, even actions you realize you wouldn't need to, like cutting, risky sex, negligent driving, and alcohol consumption. You could even believe that there is no other option.

Changing your conduct from being under your control to being in charge. It's critical to understand that these spontaneous actions have a purpose. These are coping strategies for handling stress. Even if only momentarily, they improve your mood. Yet, the overall expenses are rather significant.

Learning to handle suffering is the first step toward regaining control over your conduct. It is essential for altering BPD's harmful tendencies.

You'll be able to stop yourself from acting out if you possess the capacity to withstand suffering. You would discover how to navigate through challenging feelings while regaining the security of the situation rather than responding to them with self-destructive actions.

Although the tools will instruct you on how to manage discomfort, it goes further. Also, it will show you how to get from feeling mentally shuttered to completely feeling your thoughts. Whenever you try to suppress bad sensations, you are also prevented from experiencing the entire spectrum of happy emotions like pleasure, serenity, and satisfaction. This enables you to feel all of these. A workout to assist you to center yourself and restore grip

There is no way to "imagine oneself" calm after the combat response has been activated. Consider concentrating on your physical sensations rather than your thoughts. The grounding practice that follows is a quick, easy approach to stop being impulsive, calm down, and restore control. In only a few short minutes, it may have a significant impact.

Choose a peaceful area and take a seat comfortably.

Concentrate on the sensations you are having in your body. Feel the floor where you are seated. Feel the ground under your feet. On your lap, feel your hands. Take calm, breathing exercises while focusing on your respiration. Inhale gently. Let's pause for three counts. Then exhale gently, waiting again for a third count. This can be done for a some minutes. In an emergency, divert your attention. Jarring oneself may assist if your efforts to chill out a bit aren't succeeding and you're feeling pressured by harmful desires. What you need to do is to divert your attention long sufficient to make the unpleasant inclination pass. Anything that catches your interest can serve, but distraction works best once the task is also relaxing.

Furthermore to the consciousness tactics outlined earlier, consider the following:

Watch Netflix. Select an activity that is opposed to how you are feeling: a joke if you are sad, or whatever calming if you are furious or irritated.

Choose something you like that will keep you occupied. Landscaping, sketching, playing musical instruments, crocheting, sitting down, playing a video game, or performing a Crossword or word challenge are all examples.

Put yourself on task. You may also divert yourself by cleaning your house, performing yard work, going shopping and cooking, primping your companion, or carrying out the washing.

Start moving. Exercising vigorously is a great method to have your blood running and blow off steam. If you're feeling anxious, try some soothing hobbies like meditation or a stroll around your block.

Make a phone call to a buddy. Chatting with anyone you confide in may be an accurate product approach to divert yourself, feel much better, and get clarity.

Develop your self-confidence. You've undoubtedly battled to establish stable, rewarding relationships with lovers, colleagues, and acquaintances if you have a borderline personality disorder. This could be because you have difficulty taking a step back and viewing things in a different light from others. You tend to misinterpret people's thoughts and emotions, to misinterpret how others perceive you, and to disregard how your behavior affects others. It doesn't mean you do not care, but you have a massive blind spot when it comes to certain other people. The first step is to recognize your interpersonal blind spot. After you stop trying to blame others, you may begin to work on improving your connections with others and your social abilities.

Examine your preconceptions.

When you're distracted by anxiety and pessimism, as individuals with BPD frequently are, it is indeed easy to misinterpret others' intentions. Examine your preconceptions if you are aware of this propensity. Keep in mind that you're not a good judge of character! Consider some other reasons before taking a step of leaping to (typically uncompromising) judgments. As an example, suppose your spouse was harsh with you over the phone, which has left you feeling uneasy and concerned that they've stopped being interested in you. Before acting on your feelings:

Spend some time studying the many options. Perhaps your spouse is under stress at work. Maybe he's experiencing a difficult day. Perhaps he hasn't yet taken his coffee. There are some possible explanations for his reactions.

Request that the individual clarify their objectives. Asking another individual what it is they're experiencing or thinking is among the simplest methods to test your assumptions. Check to see if they meant what they said or did. Instead of asking accusatorial questions, try a gentler tone: "I might be mistaken, but it feels like..." or "Maybe I'm being unduly emotional, but..."

Put an end to illusion.

Do you have the propensity to transfer your bad emotions onto other people? When you're feeling down about yourself, do you strike out at others? Do you consider comments or suggestions for improvement to be a direct insult? If this is the case, you may be experiencing projection issues.

You must learn to put the brakes on to combat projection, just as you did to control your impulsive actions. Pay attention to your feelings and your body's physical experiences. Keep an eye out for symptoms of stress including a racing heartbeat, tense muscles, perspiration, nausea, or dizziness. While you're in this mood, you'll probably launch through an assault and utter which you'll come to regret. Take a few calm, deep breaths while pausing. then pose the following three queries to yourself:

Am I mad at myself?

Is this shame or fear I'm experiencing?

Am I afraid of being left behind?

Pause from talking if the response is affirmative. To continue the conversation, let the other person know that you need some time to collect your thoughts since you're feeling emotional.

Accept accountability for your part.

Ultimately, it's critical to accept accountability for your part in the connections you maintain. Consider how your behavior may be causing issues. What emotions do your actions and words evoke in your loved ones? Are you making the mistake of assuming that the other person is either completely nice or completely bad? You'll start to see a change in the caliber of your relationships when you take the opportunity to envision yourself in other words —, to give others the benefit of the skepticism, and to lower your dismissiveness.

CHAPTER 3

Figuring out the egotist

Frequently jealous, vainglorious, lacking sympathy, manipulative, entitled, and frantic for consideration and reverence, egomaniacs can make our lives troublesome and testing. They are additionally befuddling.

While sitting with a self-absorbed patient, I should set myself up to tune in past the words or records they give to tune into a mysterious universe of passing changes of points, unexpected unobtrusive glints of feeling, and sudden yet unsaid shifts in the manner in which my patient is connecting with me. These movements and redirections, which signal basic agony, are by and large happening inside the setting of self-swelling stories, alongside protests about others, including me. Because of clinical encounters in treating self-absorbed patients, coming up next are rules and exhortations to assist you with grasping the impossible-to-miss mental universe of the egotist.

Instructions to Deal with an Egotist

You might contemplate whether your accomplice, colleague, or relative is an egotist. While many individuals have what specialists call egotistical qualities, similar to grandiosity and privilege (believing they're owed something), individuals determined to have the self-involved behavioral condition can be a greater test.

Having an egotist in your life can be disappointing and genuinely testing. Your relationship might rotate around them. You might feel judged and depleted by their demands. Growing up with this profoundly controlling individual was very difficult.

How to Recognize an Egomaniac

Egomaniacs have serious areas of strength and pretentiousness. That implies they believe they're a higher priority than others and frequently search out profound respect.

Egotists often: Have a solid feeling of pomposity (they have elevated degrees of confidence, grandiosity, and fearlessness, and frequently feel like they're better than others)

- Are presumptuous
- Exploit others to get what they need
- Accept they're extraordinary or unique
- Misrepresent accomplishments and abilities
- Need steady esteem
- Feel envy toward others
- Accept others envy them
- Need compassion
- Are fixated on dreams of splendor, power, or achievement
- Have a feeling of entitlement Narcissists and Connections

Egomaniacs might take the necessary steps to get what they need. They by and large don't feel empathy and can't interface personally with others, even individuals who are nearest to them.

At work, an egotist might look for reverence, regardless of whether it harms others. They might assume acknowledgment for others' work, subvert associates, or change their way of behaving to get the endorsement from more significant level individuals. They might appear to be well-disposed and diligent, however, there's something else to it besides what meets the eye. Sometimes it's ideal to cut attaches with an egotist, particularly on the off chance that they're oppressive.

Find these ways to deal with an egotist:

Educate yourself. Figure out more about the confusion. It can assist you with figuring out the egotist's assets and shortcomings and figuring out how to deal with them better. Knowing what their identity is may likewise permit you to acknowledge what is happening for what it is and have practical assumptions.

Make limits. Be clear about your limits. It might disturb or dishearten the egomaniac, yet at the same that is Completely fine. Keep in mind, you must get a grip on that individual's feelings. Speak up for yourself. At the point when you want something, be clear and compact. Ensure they comprehend your solicitation.

Watch your phrasing. Egotists don't take productive analysis well. Attempt to offer remarks in cautious, positive ways.

Remain cool-headed. Do whatever it takes not to respond if they attempt to start a ruckus for no obvious reason or gaslight you (making you question your existence). On the off chance that they suddenly erupt, consider them a 3-year-old who feels dismissed because their parent sets a sleep time. Create an emotionally supportive network. Living with an egotist can prompt sensations of weakness, disarray, and self-question. Ensure you have a center gathering in your life that can uphold you.

Get a guide. Treatment won't fix your accomplice's self-centeredness, however, it might take care of your work-specific things. This can show you ways of moving toward critical thinking with the egomaniac.

How Not to Manage an Egomaniac

Certain things might set off issues with an egomaniac, so it's ideal to keep away from them. Don't contend or stand up to. It's best not to straightforwardly face an egotist. As troublesome as it could be to continually sneak around them, it tends to be smarter to deal with their need to feel in control.

Try not to attempt to guide them. Egomaniacs like to have control and frequently dread losing it. Endeavors to lead or teach an egotist will frequently come up short.

Try not to anticipate that they should see your perspective. Egotists could do without conceding when they're off-base or that they're repulsive, so attempting to make them see things your way could backfire. Don't anticipate profound, significant correspondence. Egotists have almost no compassion, so legit, genuine correspondence frequently doesn't traverse and could make an unexpected eruption of fury or closure reaction.

Try not to go over previous issues. Try not to attempt to make them see a long queue of conduct going back years - - or how they're very much like their dad for instance. All things being equal, remain in the current when you express demands or are put in a horrible mood.

Individuals with a self-centered behavioral condition as a rule don't change, so remember that. Regardless of whether you figure out how to deal with your relationship better, it likely will not at any point be a sound relationship.

Causes of Clandestine Selfishness

The specific reasons for incognito self-absorption are not completely perceived, however, all things considered, various variables contribute. Specialists recommend that self-centered behavioral condition is connected to factors including:

- Hereditary qualities
- Adolescence misuse and injury
- Childhood and associations with parental figures
- Character and temperament

One investigation discovered that individuals with the self-absorbed behavioral condition are bound to have grown up with guardians who were exceptionally centered around status and achievements. Because they were frequently caused to feel better than different youngsters, the conviction that they are unique and more significant than others might endure into adulthood.

It isn't clear, be that as it may, why an egotistical way of behaving is once in a while shown in clandestine as opposed to obvious ways. A few circumstances that could set off an incognito egomaniac include:

- Being overlooked
- Feeling affronted
- Dangers to their inner self
- Sensations of disgrace
- Being around high-status individuals
- Feeling less alluring or less instructed than others
- Having less of something than others
- Not standing out they assume they merit
- Envy
- Absence of control.

The most effective method to Manage an Incognito Egotist

You may at present be in an individual relationship with a clandestine egotist, whether it be a relative, colleague, or critical other. Even though you have no control over what an egotist does, you have some control over how you act and collaborate with them. There are steps that you can take to shield yourself from clandestine self-involved misuse.

Try not to Think about It Literally
While managing an egomaniac, whether secret or obvious, their manipulative way of behaving can feel extremely private. The absence of respect, disposition for narcissism, examples of control, and misleading ways of behaving can feel extremely private when on the less-than-desirable end.

Regardless of how difficult the ways of behaving could feel at the time, it's memorable's essential that they don't have anything to do with you.
An egotist acts in regrettable ways due to something unfortunate inside them — not because there is an undesirable thing about them.

It is alright to take a gander at the circumstance and the cooperation as to how you add to them. In any case, it is vital while managing an egomaniac that you let them "own" their part. Egomaniacs believe you should think about it literally because that is the way they keep up with influence. Keep in mind, an egotist feels little, so they need to make themselves "enormous" in some way or another.

Put down Stopping points
Egotists don't have sound boundaries. Because secret egomaniacs need compassion, have areas of strength for qualification, and take advantage of others, limits are something that impedes their objectives. The more you can work on defining limits with an egotist, the more reliably you are passing on to them that their strategies are not working.

Defining limits can be extremely challenging, especially with an egomaniac. Recall that limits are only a way for you to let another person understand what your qualities are. Consider what is essential to you, and what your qualities are, and attempt to make limits to help them.

Understanding the reason why you are defining specific limits can assist you with having more trust in laying out them and can keep you on target assuming somebody endeavors to abuse or negligence your limits.

Advocate for Yourself

While cooperating with an incognito egomaniac, losing your voice can be simple. Since the examples of connection are so manipulative, it might require investment for you to understand that you're not upholding for yourself.

Set aside some margin to tune back in with yourself, what your identity is, and what you are about. Consider your qualities, your objectives, and your gifts. Reinforcing your relationship with yourself is key to having the option to shout out during communications with an egotist.

While pushing for yourself, the egotist has an opportunity to meet the piece of you that knows and learned of their strategies, making it less engaging for them to continue to attempt those things with you.

Make a Solid Distance

Being involved with a secretive egomaniac can feel disappointing and overpowering. There are times when it very well may be hard to make the distance between you and that individual, for example, with a relative or colleague.

Restricting individual collaborations, requesting to be moved to an alternate area in your office, enjoying reprieves at an alternate time, or removing contact may be what is essential on the off chance that you are being wounded by somebody's self-absorption. The objective of making distance isn't to harm the other individual; the objective is to safeguard yourself and make space for you to recuperate.

CHAPTER 4

Living in a strain cooker as a marginal behavioral condition patient

Living with marginal behavioral condition (BPD) can be tested and it might some of the time want to live in a tension cooker. Individuals with BPD frequently battle with extreme and unsound feelings, indiscreet ways of behaving, and troubles with connections. This are a few idea that might be useful:

Look for proficient assistance: It's critical to work with emotional well-being proficient who is prepared in treating BPD. A specialist can assist you with mastering abilities to deal with your feelings, adapt to pressure, and work on your connections.

Practice care: Care is a method that can assist you with zeroing in on the current second and lessen pressure. You can rehearse care by taking full breaths, noticing your contemplations without judgment, and zeroing in on your faculties.

Foster solid survival techniques: Take part in exercises that you appreciate, like activity, workmanship, or music. Try not to utilize medications or liquor to adapt to troublesome feelings, as they can deteriorate BPD side effects.

Construct an encouraging group of people: Interface with loved ones who can offer close-to-home help. Join a care group for individuals with BPD, which can give a feeling of local area and approval.

Deal with yourself: It's critical to focus on taking care of oneself, like getting sufficient rest, eating a sound eating routine, and participating in exercises that encourage you.
Recall that recuperation from BPD is conceivable with the right treatment and backing. It might require investment and exertion, yet with tirelessness and persistence, you can figure out how to deal with your side effects and lead a satisfying life.

CHAPTER 5

Grasp your circumstances: defining limits and improving abilities

Practice mindfulness: Focus on your viewpoints, sentiments, and ways of behaving to acquire knowledge about your responses to various circumstances.

Ponder previous encounters: Consider how you've taken care of comparative circumstances before and what you can gain from those encounters.

Look for criticism: Ask confided-in companions or relatives for their point of view on your conduct in specific circumstances.
Recognize your qualities: Figure out what is essential to you and what you endlessly won't endure in your connections and associations with others.

Convey your limits: Obviously and deferentially impart your limits to other people.
Uphold your limits: Be reliable in implementing your limits, regardless of whether it's troublesome or awkward.

Recognize regions for development: Evaluate your assets and shortcomings and distinguish regions where you might want to move along.

Search our assets: Make the most of instructive open doors, like studios, classes, or online courses, to foster new abilities.

Practice consistently: Customary practice can assist you with dominating new abilities and making them a piece of your day-to-day daily schedule.

Recollect that grasping your circumstances, defining limits, and leveling up abilities is a continuous interaction. With constancy and responsibility, you can gain ground and accomplish more prominent mindfulness, better connections, and self-awareness

CHAPTER 6

Making a security plan

Making a well-being plan can be a significant piece of overseeing marginal behavioral condition (BPD) and remaining protected during seasons of emergency. Here are moves toward making a security plan:

Recognize triggers: Make a rundown of circumstances, occasions, or individuals that might set off serious feelings or troubling considerations.

Make a rundown of survival methods: Distinguish solid survival techniques that can assist you with dealing with your feelings during seasons of pressure or emergency. Models might incorporate profound breathing activities, going for a stroll, or conversing with a confided-in companion or relative.

Distinguish steady individuals: Make a rundown of individuals who you can go to for consistent reassurance, for example, a specialist, an emergency hotline, or a confided-in companion or relative.

Foster an emergency plan: Distinguish steps you can take during an emergency to guard yourself, for example, reaching an emergency helpline or going to the trauma center.

Make an arrangement for after an emergency: Recognize taking care of oneself procedures that can assist you with dealing with your feelings after an emergency, for example, getting some much-needed rest work or participating in exercises that you appreciate.

Survey and update your arrangement consistently: Audit your well-being plan routinely and make refreshes depending on the situation because of changes in your psychological well-being, triggers, methods for dealing with especially difficult times, or an emotionally supportive network.

Recall that making a well-being plan is only one device in overseeing BPD. It's vital to work with an emotional wellness proficient who can assist you with fostering an exhaustive treatment plan that incorporates treatment, prescription, and different methodologies to deal with your side effects and work on your satisfaction.

How does a Security Plan work?

The initial step is recognizing cautioning signs. These are any encounters, feelings, considerations, or activities that might flag that an emergency is created sooner rather than later.

Even though everybody's admonition signs might be unique, I will give a couple of guides to make you think:

Feeling forlorn, not getting sufficient rest, neglecting to take medicine, feeling dismissed, getting a terrible grade, contending with a friend or family member, not eating enough, considerations stuck on repeat...

In the wake of recognizing your advance notice signs, list your inward survival techniques.

Inward survival techniques are things that you can do on your own that might divert you, assist you with feeling quite a bit improved, or take care of the issue.

Inward survival techniques might include: profound breathing, getting a tidbit, taking a walk, doing yoga, perusing a book, writing in a diary, cooking, singing or paying attention to music, sitting in front of the television, painting, and utilizing my DBT skills.

You may likewise incorporate your emergency unit (more on that underneath) in your interior ways of dealing with hardship or stress.

The more inner survival methods you have, the better. Try not to restrict yourself to the 3 on the layout if you have more.

Including others in your Wellbeing Plan

There are three different ways we include others in the well-being plan:

1. Interruptions - individuals who we may not be guaranteed to feel open to offering to, yet who can divert us. Perhaps you ask a neighbor how their day is going, or request that a companion watch a Netflix show with you.
Having individuals who give interruption can assist you with keeping your psyche off the emergency until it passes, or until better assistance shows up.

2. Individuals you can request help - these are individuals who are not experts, but rather who you can call when you truly need support.
Perhaps these are companions, relatives, or accomplices, who have communicated an interest in your psychological prosperity or well-being.
If it's not too much trouble, note that the job of these individuals isn't to work you out of an emergency - individuals in this part may be simply sufficiently lucid to help you to remember the abilities you have, or associate

you with the assets you want at that time, or drive you to an arrangement that you want.

3. **Experts or offices you can contact during an emergency** - this is where you will put your specialist as well as a therapist if you have them.

This is likewise where you will put your nearby emotional well-being emergency line.

To find your nearby emotional well-being emergency line, google your city/region/state name (contingent upon where you reside, the administrations might be given at an alternate level) in addition to the words "psychological well-being emergency."

Making the climate safe

This will be different for everybody; it will rely upon what you want to keep up with security.

This generally implies ensuring that guns, different weapons, and possibly hazardous prescriptions are eliminated from the home. It might include avoiding potential risk. Suggestions such as breaking new ground here can be advice able. Do you have to erase specific online entertainment applications for a brief timeframe to be protected? Do you want space away from specific individuals? Is it useful to have pets with you? Consider whatever would make the climate pretty much protected, and make a note of it here.

What makes daily routine worth experiencing?

At the actual lower part of the security plan is a line that says "the one thing that means quite a bit to me and worth living for is:____"
Record this ahead of time, since minds are entertaining here and there. At the point when you are in an emergency, your mind might let you know that nothing merits living for - so recording it before the emergency is significant.
What is important to you? What dreams do you have for your future? Are there individuals or creatures who you need to see develop? Do you have objectives you want to wrap up? What's on your list of must-dos?

Emergency Unit

An emergency unit is an actual pack - like a case or a sack - that you set up ahead of an emergency.

It contains things that can assist you with mitigating yourself when you are heightened. Put the most that you would be able - or make separate ones (for instance, one for home, and a convenient one for school/work/the vehicle).

You can assemble the emergency unit with a friend or family member, and you can request that your cherished one remind you about the emergency pack when you want.

You can incorporate anything that assists you with feeling quite a bit improved, yet here is an aide of interesting points:

1. Temperature - I energetically suggest putting one of those moments ice packs in your emergency unit. You can break it when you are in an emergency and hold it over your face for roughly 30 seconds. This makes an actual reaction in the body that dials back emergency considerations.

You may likewise need to consider something warm, similar to a warming cushion or a warm cover, assuming you feel that sounds mitigating.

2. Suggestions to self - think of yourself confident notes and put them in the emergency pack. Brief yourself to utilize the abilities you now have, yet may disregard them while in an emergency (incorporate directions if you want). Take a stab at utilizing brilliantly shaded notecards, or compose the updates in beautiful ink or block letters.

3. Feeling of smell - what fragrances do you track down quieting? Might you at any point get a body moisturizer, light, or chapstick in those fragrances? The antiperspirant, fragrance, or body wash of an individual who encourages you?

4. Feeling of touch - plush toys, delicate covers or hoodies, weighted covers, a twirly gig, play batter, a recuperating gem, stress balls - anything that you can contact or grasp that feels unwinding to you.

5. Innovativeness - put a notepad, workmanship supplies, or anything instruments you want to make your specialty. On the off chance that your device doesn't squeeze into the crate (ex: if you express imagination by singing), compose a suggestion to yourself on a notecard and put that in the case.

6. Feeling of taste/glucose - tasting our number one food varieties can alleviate. Furthermore, when we are ravenous, we are all the more genuinely dysregulated. Put a few durable delectable tidbits or home-grown tea in your emergency pack.

7. Pictures - print out pictures of pets, friends and family, most loved spots, or things you seek from here on out.

8. Feeling of sound - commotion dropping earphones for assuming you are over-animated. A playlist of tunes that are consoling. ASMR recordings or digital broadcasts.

9. Idealism - do you have a most loved book that you can lose all sense of direction in? A computer game? A DVD of your #1 film?

10. Interruptions - a book of word riddles or Sudoku. Doing rationale issues or riddles powers the mind out of feeling mode and into rational mode.

Utilizing the Wellbeing Plan and Emergency Unit

Ensure you put the Security Plan and Emergency Pack together ahead of time! It accomplishes take a little work and imaginative reasoning, and it is difficult to do it while you are in an emergency.

Put the Wellbeing Plan report itself in a noticeable/open spot, so you generally approach it. Share it with steady friends and family.

If you maintain that a friend or family member should be a piece of your Security Plan, check in with them. Ensure that they are capable and ready to do what you request (model, it probably won't be workable for somebody who lives far away to visit you, yet perhaps they can FaceTime you).

Urge your friends and family to remind you to utilize your arrangement - and let them know how you need to be reminded. Enable your adored one to tell you when they think you are in an emergency - even though meeting at the time may be terrible. Concur ahead of time the way that you believe those discussions should go.

It very well might be useful to have a code word with your friends and family, similar to, "I'm having the Large Miserable, could you at any point assist me with my arrangement."

For example, "When I lack the zeal, it would be useful on the off chance that you proceeded to get the get well plan for me off the cooler, however, I need to sort out which adapting abilities to utilize." or on the other hand "Assuming I appear as though I'm in an emergency, if it's not too much trouble, utilize our code word as opposed to letting me know I want to quiet down."

Most importantly,

What makes a well-being arrangement and an emergency pack work, is whether you are willing and ready to utilize them when you want. Set a focus on making it individual to you, so that when the opportunity arrives, you need to utilize it.

Life merits living.

Adapting to terrible times.

You could have times when everything appears an excessive amount to adapt to and you feel very bothered. This is called having an emergency.

If you see well-being experts during an emergency, they will zero in on the 'present time and place'. An emergency isn't the most ideal opportunity to begin a top-to-bottom conversation about previous encounters or relationship issues. It is normally better for you to think about those issues later during your standard treatment with your principal treatment supplier.

In any event, when you are major areas of strength for encountering, you ought to remain associated with tracking down answers to your concerns. This implies individuals who are treating you for your BPD won't pursue every one of your choices for you. They will ask you for your thoughts and anticipate that you should participate in making arrangements to recover.

Intending to guard yourself

Have an arrangement for what to do when you feel in an emergency - what should be done to guard yourself, including when to contact crisis administrations. This sort of plan is here and there called a well-being plan.

A security plan assists you with thinking obviously when you are troubled. At the point when you are well, and with the assistance of your treatment supplier, you ought to record an arrangement that you can follow when you want it. You can likewise give a duplicate to your accomplice or family.

Ask the principal well-being proficient who gets your BPD to work with you to make a security arrangement. It ought to be remembered for your administration plan as a unique segment.

Data that ought to be in your well-being plan

Your objectives for treatment and issues that you are dealing with, including a rundown of transient objectives and long-haul objectives.

Circumstances that cause you to feel dangerous or upset to the point of causing an emergency.

Things that you can do to get past an emergency - these could be methodologies that you have utilized before that have helped you get by and won't hurt you.

Things that you shouldn't do during an emergency - list things that you have attempted before an emergency that didn't work or compounded the situation.

Things that your accomplice or family can accomplish for you that will help you.

Individuals you can contact for help during an emergency - list telephone quantities of individuals who support you (for example your accomplice or a relative, your therapist, case manager, school guide, GP) or associations that can help (for example Lifesaver, crisis benefits, a psychological well-being line).

CHAPTER 7

What happens next? Settling on conclusions about your relationship as a fringe and self-involved BPD

Coming to conclusions about connections can be especially trying for people with the marginal behavioral condition (BPD) and self-centered behavioral condition (NPD) because of troubles with feeling guidelines and relational working. Here are a few ways to come to conclusions about your relationship:

Look for proficient assistance: It's vital to work with emotional well-being proficient who is prepared in treating BPD and NPD. A specialist can assist you with acquiring an understanding of your examples of conduct in connections and foster abilities to work on your correspondence, profound guideline, and survival methods.

Assess the relationship: Think about the positive and negative parts of the relationship, and assess whether it's gathering your requirements and adding to your general prosperity.

Put down stopping points: Recognize your limits and impart them obviously to your accomplice. Limits can assist you with keeping a feeling of control and diminish sensations of overpowering in the relationship.

Practice taking care of oneself: Focus on taking care of oneself exercises that assist you with dealing with your feelings and lessen pressure. This might incorporate activity, care, investing energy with steady loved ones, or participating in leisure activities or interests that you appreciate.

Think about the effect on your psychological wellness: Assess what the relationship is meaning for your emotional well-being and whether it's adding to the side effects of BPD or NPD. On the off chance that the relationship is having an adverse consequence, taking into account finishing it might be essential.

Recollect that settling on conclusions about connections can be intricate and close to home, and moving toward these choices with care and thoughtfulness is significant. With the assistance of an emotional well-being proficiency and a pledge to take care of oneself and limit setting, people with BPD and NPD can work on their connections and accomplish more prominent profound security and prosperity.

Step-by-step instructions to help you collaborate with BPD

You and your accomplice might have learned various ways to deal with adoration, which can introduce one-of-a-kind learning potential and open doors for you two.

Remembering that a portion of your accomplice's ways of behaving is not an individual decision, but rather a side effect, may assist you with keeping things in context.

It's exceptionally fitting that you likewise center around your feelings, psychological wellness, and individual security. Their eagerness to chip away at dealing with their side effects now has nothing to do with you.

Proficient help can help, however, the individual must settle on the choice to look for help.

Where you 'stand' may move

While you're dating somebody with BPD, times, when you might go from, are being the legend to being the lowlife in their eyes.

This is designated "parting," a side effect where you're seen as either completely fine or all terrible. It's occasionally a response to profound agony. To oversee it, they might have to make you the "miscreant" for some time.

Your accomplice might try and make the additional stride and request a break.

This doesn't guarantee to mean they couldn't care less about you. They might be struggling with expressing feelings, or they might be dreading you leaving, so it feels more straightforward to cut off the friendship before you do.

You might find it supportive to give them space to chill off and demand that you return to the discussion sometime in the not-too-distant future, to get clearness on where you stand.

Consolation might be fundamental

You might find that your accomplice needs more consolation than you do.

Research Trusted Source demonstrates the way that living with marginal character can make it challenging to believe that individuals won't leave.

Your accomplice might invest a ton of energy searching for pieces of information about how you feel, such as examining instant messages, ruminating over discussions, or testing you.

You might be approached to give additional consolation through your words, activities, or actual warmth.

At the point when it feels regular, it's smart to straightforwardly communicate how you feel as frequently as possible.

Responses might require a clarification

At times the people who live with BPD can hyper-read the room.

One test with this, however, is that they might detect something in your looks or manner of speaking that you won't be guaranteed to feel or that may not be related to them.

For instance, your accomplice might think you look exhausted and close you're not content with them. You may be including the tip for the bill in your mind.

Realize that your accomplice might request that you explain your looks, manner of speaking, or messages frequently to ensure that you're seeing one another.

You may likewise confront a few false impressions, so it's really smart to try not to get cautious when your accomplice misreads you. Explanation and consolation will go far while dating somebody with marginal character.

Objectives might move and change and It could be hard for your accomplice to work at a specific employment where they feel tested, reprimanded, or dismissed. Truth be told, it shows that they may imprudently stop, or cut attaches with significant associations, and afterward think twice about it.

Realizing this early can assist you two with planning for what's in store. You might need to examine an investment account or a contingency plan, so you're adjusted concerning funds.

Online entertainment might be a presence

It has been found that the individuals who live with BPD might utilize web-based entertainment more than the people who don't, maybe for approval and consolation.

Its been found that certain individuals may unexpectedly remove others, such as unfriending or obstructing them. Make an effort not to think about it assuming that your accomplice does this to you seemingly out of the blue.

Additionally, if you feel like you're contending with your accomplice's telephone, request what you want. For instance, a solicitation to have supper quite recently you two, sans screens.

You may likewise find that communicating your appreciation in web-based entertainment might cause them to have a solid sense of reassurance in the relationship. Assuming this is the sort of thing that feels alright with you, take a stab at posting photographs together or adding heartfelt remarks to what they post.

Instructions to fortify your bond

There are a few different ways you can reinforce your organization by cooperating on a couple of systems.

Pay attention to comprehend

You experienced passionate feelings for this individual which is as it should be. In any event, during troublesome minutes, recollect what that is. Learn. Teach yourself. Be that as it may, in particular, be a decent audience. Contemplate everything that your accomplice is attempting to say to you, under their feelings and ways of behaving. Ask yourself, what are their expectations?

If you meet them where they are, as opposed to attempting to change them to meet you where you will be, you will want to advance more straightforwardly together, "Approve and recognize, regardless of whether you concur."

You may likewise need to consider communicating should be paid attention to and empowering your accomplice to twofold check before expecting how you feel.

Further, develop your relational abilities

Powerful correspondence takes work, yet the paste keeps your relationship intact. You might find it helpful to:

70

record what you need to say and request that your accomplice do likewise
take full breaths before you talk
center around each issue in turn
keep open non-verbal communication
use "I" articulations
Additionally, go ahead and pump the brakes. At the point when we answer naturally to feelings, we will more often than not do and make statements that we could later lament. "On the off chance that you feel like things are beginning to get warmed among you and your accomplice, take a 'break' and return once you've both chilled a little."
Enroll the assistance of a couple's specialist
Couples treatment can make a protected and unbiased space to communicate your sentiments and concerns,
A couple's specialist can direct you by posing the right inquiries and assist the two players with feeling comprehended and heard. The specialist can go on to teach, and back you up as you make progress toward a more conducive and sound relationship.

CONCLUSION

At the point when you travel to another nation, realize the neighborhood customs are significant. While you're collaborating with somebody with BPD, it's significant to comprehend that their oblivious presumptions might be altogether different from yours. They might include: I should be adored by every one of the notable individuals in my day-to-day existence consistently or, in all likelihood I'm useless. I should be totally skillful in all ways to be an advantageous individual. Certain individuals are great and every little thing about them is awesome. Others are completely terrible and ought to be faulted and rebuffed for it. My sentiments are brought about by outer occasions. I have zero power over my feelings or the things I do in response to them. No one thinks often about me however much I care about them, so I lose everybody I care about — in spite of the frantic things I do to prevent them from leaving me. On the off chance that somebody mistreats me, I become terrible. Basically, individuals with BPD shift their focus over to others to deal with their affection for them. Somebody with BPD believes that others should give them things they view as challenging to supply for themselves, like self-esteem, stable mindsets, and a feeling of personality. In particular, they are looking for a sustaining guardian whose endless love and sympathy will fill the dark opening of void and misery inside them. Individuals with BPD attempt to deal with their aggravation through their connections with others. As we have made sense of, projections, seethes, analysis, accusing, and other protection instruments might be endeavors to inspire you to sympathize with their aggravation for them. At the point when you self-assuredly divert the aggravation back to the individual with BPD so they can start to manage it, you are breaking an agreement that you didn't realize you marked. Normally, the individual with BPD will view this as troubling. The individual with BPD will presumably make a countermove. This is an activity intended to reestablish things to how they were. Countermoves likewise assist individuals with supporting their activities, both to themselves and to you. This component is vital on the grounds that it appears to make the extortion adequate — even honorable. Your capacity to endure these countermoves will decide the future course of your relationship.

Playing safe always